PLANT BASED DIET FOR ATHLETES

Maximizing Athletic Performance through the
Power of Plant-Based Nutrition

Helen R. Galante

TABLE OF CONTENTS

INTRODUCTION

Definition of a plant-based diet for athletes

A plant-based diet for athletes is a dietary approach that emphasizes the consumption of whole, minimally processed plant-based foods to support athletic performance and overall health. This diet typically includes fruits, vegetables, whole grains, legumes, nuts, and seeds, and may also include some plant-based sources of protein such as tofu, tempeh, and seitan.

Athletes who follow a plant-based diet may also choose to incorporate some fortified plant-based products such as plant-based milks and protein powders to meet their specific nutritional needs.

Additionally, some athletes may choose to supplement their plant-based diet with vitamin B12, iron, and other nutrients that are typically found in animal-based foods.

Research has shown that a plant-based diet can provide sufficient amounts of protein, carbohydrates, and healthy fats to support athletic performance and recovery. It may also offer additional health benefits such as improved cardiovascular health, reduced inflammation, and better glycemic control. However, athletes following a plant-based diet should ensure they are meeting their specific nutritional needs to support their training and competition demands. It is recommended that athletes work with a registered dietitian to develop a well-planned and balanced plant-based diet that meets their individual needs.

Benefits of a plant-based diet for athletes

Plant-based diets can offer a range of benefits for athletes, including:

Improved cardiovascular health: Plant-based diets are rich in fiber, vitamins, minerals, and antioxidants, which can help to lower cholesterol levels and reduce the risk of heart disease.

Faster recovery: Plant-based diets are often rich in anti-inflammatory foods, such as fruits, vegetables, nuts, and seeds, which can help to reduce inflammation in the body and speed up recovery after exercise.

Increased energy and stamina: Plant-based diets can provide the body with the necessary carbohydrates, vitamins, and minerals needed for sustained energy throughout the day and during athletic performance.

Reduced risk of chronic diseases: Plant-based diets have been linked to a reduced risk of chronic diseases, such as diabetes, cancer, and obesity, which can negatively impact athletic performance.

Improved digestion: Plant-based diets are often rich in fiber, which can improve digestion and prevent gastrointestinal issues that may interfere with athletic performance.

Reduced inflammation: Plant-based diets can help to reduce inflammation in the body, which can improve overall health and reduce the risk of injury.

Improved mental health: Plant-based diets have been linked to improved mood and reduced stress levels, which can be beneficial for athletes who often face high levels of stress and pressure.

Overall, plant-based diets can provide athletes with the necessary nutrients and energy needed to perform at their best while also improving their overall health and reducing the risk of injury and chronic diseases.

Common misconceptions about plant-based diets and athletic performance

There are several common misconceptions about plant-based diets and athletic performance. Here are a few:

Plant-based diets don't provide enough protein: Many people believe that it is difficult to get enough protein on a plant-based diet. However, this is a misconception. There are many plant-based sources of protein, including lentils, beans, tofu, tempeh, seitan, nuts, and seeds. These foods can provide all the amino acids needed for muscle building and repair.

Plant-based diets are low in energy: Another misconception is that plant-based diets are low in energy and can lead to fatigue and decreased athletic performance. However, plant-based diets can be just as energy-dense as meat-based diets, and with proper planning, athletes can consume enough calories to fuel their workouts.

Plant-based diets don't provide enough nutrients: Some people believe that plant-based diets don't provide enough nutrients, such as iron, calcium, and vitamin B12. However, with careful planning and attention to food choices, it is possible to get all the necessary nutrients from a plant-based diet.

Plant-based diets are not suitable for building muscle: Many people believe that animal protein is necessary for building muscle and that plant-based diets are not suitable for bodybuilding. However, plant-based sources of protein can be just as effective as animal protein for muscle building, and studies have shown that plant-based diets can support muscle growth and strength.

Plant-based diets are too restrictive: Finally, some people believe that plant-based diets are too restrictive and limit food choices, making it difficult to meet their nutritional needs. However, with the wide variety of plant-based foods available, it is possible to create a balanced and diverse diet that meets all nutritional needs.

CHAPTER ONE

The Nutritional Needs of Athletes

Athletes have unique nutritional needs that vary based on their sport, training intensity, body size, and goals. Adequate nutrition is essential for optimal athletic performance, endurance, and recovery. Here are some key nutrients and dietary recommendations for athletes:

Carbohydrates: Carbohydrates are the primary source of energy for athletes. They should make up at least 50% of an athlete's daily calorie intake. Good sources of carbohydrates include whole grains, fruits, vegetables, and legumes.

Protein: Protein is important for muscle growth and repair. Athletes should aim for 1.2-2.0 grams of protein per kilogram of body weight per day, depending on their training level. Good sources of protein include lean meats, fish, eggs, dairy products, and plant-based sources such as legumes, tofu, and tempeh.

Fats: Fats are essential for energy production and hormone regulation. Athletes should aim for 20-35% of their daily calorie intake to come from healthy fats such as nuts, seeds, avocados, olive oil, and fatty fish.

Hydration: Athletes should drink plenty of fluids before, during, and after exercise to maintain hydration. Water is usually sufficient for most athletes, but for intense exercise lasting longer than an hour, sports drinks that contain electrolytes may be necessary.

Vitamins and Minerals: Athletes require adequate amounts of vitamins and minerals to support their immune system, energy production, and muscle function. A balanced diet rich in fruits, vegetables, whole grains, lean protein, and healthy fats should provide sufficient amounts of vitamins and minerals. However, athletes may need to supplement with specific nutrients if they have deficiencies or have increased nutrient needs due to their training.

Athletes require a balanced diet that provides sufficient amounts of carbohydrates, protein, fats, vitamins, and minerals to support their performance and recovery. It's important to consult a registered dietitian or sports nutritionist to determine individualized nutrient needs and recommendations.

Macronutrient needs for athletes

Athletes have increased nutrient requirements due to the demands placed on their bodies during training and competition. Macronutrients are the nutrients required in larger amounts and include carbohydrates, protein, and fat. Here are the recommended macronutrient needs for athletes:

Carbohydrates: Carbohydrates are the primary source of energy for athletes. They are stored in the muscles and liver as glycogen and are used during exercise. Athletes should aim to consume 6-10 grams of carbohydrates per kilogram of body weight per day, with higher amounts needed for endurance athletes.

Protein: Protein is important for building and repairing muscle tissue. Athletes should aim to consume 1.2-2 grams of protein per kilogram of body weight per day, with higher amounts needed for strength and power athletes.

Fat: Fat is a source of energy during prolonged exercise and also plays a role in hormone production and cell function. Athletes should aim to consume 20-30% of their total daily calories from fat.

It's important to note that individual needs may vary depending on factors such as training volume, intensity, and sport-specific requirements. It's recommended that athletes consult with a registered dietitian to develop a personalized nutrition plan that meets their individual needs.

Micronutrient needs for athletes

Micronutrients are essential vitamins and minerals required in small quantities by the body to function properly. For athletes, meeting the recommended daily intake of micronutrients is crucial for maintaining overall health, supporting immune function, and enhancing physical performance. Here are some of the essential micronutrients for athletes and their functions:

Iron: Iron is essential for transporting oxygen to the muscles, and a deficiency in iron can lead to fatigue and decreased endurance. Athletes who participate in endurance sports, such as running or cycling, may require higher levels of iron intake.

Calcium: Calcium is important for maintaining bone health, which is essential for athletes who participate in high-impact sports. Inadequate calcium intake can increase the risk of stress fractures and other bone injuries.

Vitamin D: Vitamin D plays a critical role in bone health, and it also supports immune function. Athletes who train indoors or in low sunlight areas may be at risk for vitamin D deficiency.

B-vitamins: B-vitamins are important for energy production, and they can also help to reduce inflammation and support immune function. Athletes who participate in high-intensity sports may require higher levels of B-vitamin intake.

Magnesium: Magnesium is important for muscle and nerve function, and it also plays a role in energy production. Athletes who engage in high-intensity exercise may require higher levels of magnesium intake.

Zinc: Zinc is important for immune function and wound healing, which are both critical for athletes who are at risk for injuries and infections.

It is important for athletes to consume a well-balanced diet that includes a variety of nutrient-dense foods to meet their micronutrient needs. Athletes who have specific concerns about their micronutrient intake should consult with a registered dietitian or sports nutritionist to develop an individualized nutrition plan.

How a plant-based diet can meet the nutritional needs of athletes

A plant-based diet can provide all the necessary nutrients required for athletes to maintain their performance and recover properly. Here are some ways in which a plant-based diet can meet the nutritional needs of athletes:

Carbohydrates: Plant-based foods such as fruits, vegetables, grains, and legumes are rich sources of carbohydrates that provide energy for athletes. Consuming complex carbohydrates, such as brown rice, quinoa, and sweet potatoes, can help sustain energy levels throughout the day.

Protein: While animal products are commonly thought to be the primary source of protein, there are many plant-based sources that can provide enough protein for athletes. Examples include legumes (e.g. lentils, beans, chickpeas), nuts and seeds (e.g. almonds, pumpkin seeds), soy products (e.g. tofu, tempeh), and whole grains (e.g. quinoa, amaranth). It's important to consume a variety of these protein sources to ensure that all essential amino acids are present.

Healthy Fats: Plant-based fats, such as those found in nuts, seeds, avocados, and olive oil, can provide healthy fats and omega-3 fatty acids, which are essential for brain function and reducing inflammation.

Vitamins and Minerals: Plant-based foods are rich sources of vitamins and minerals that are essential for athletes, such as vitamin C, iron, calcium, and magnesium. Leafy greens, legumes, and fortified plant milks are good sources of these nutrients.

Hydration: Adequate hydration is essential for athletes, and plant-based sources such as fruits and vegetables can help meet hydration needs. Additionally, coconut water is a natural source of electrolytes, which can be helpful for athletes during intense workouts.

A plant-based diet can provide all the necessary nutrients for athletes, as long as they consume a variety of whole foods and pay attention to meeting their nutrient needs. Working with a registered dietitian can be helpful in developing a plant-based meal plan that meets an athlete's unique needs.

CHAPTER TWO

Plant-Based Protein Sources for Athletes

There are plenty of plant-based protein sources that athletes can incorporate into their diets. Here are some options:

Legumes: Lentils, chickpeas, black beans, and kidney beans are all excellent sources of protein. They're also rich in fiber and other nutrients.

Nuts and seeds: Almonds, peanuts, pumpkin seeds, and chia seeds are all great sources of protein. They're also rich in healthy fats, which can help reduce inflammation and improve recovery.

Quinoa: This pseudo-grain is a complete protein, meaning it contains all nine essential amino acids that the body can't produce on its own.

Tofu and tempeh: These soy-based products are both rich in protein and can be used in a variety of dishes.

Seitan: This wheat-based protein is often used as a meat substitute in vegan and vegetarian dishes.

Spirulina: This blue-green algae is rich in protein and other nutrients, and can be added to smoothies or other recipes.

Vegetables: Broccoli, spinach, kale, and other leafy greens are all good sources of protein, as well as other vitamins and minerals that are important for athletic performance.

It's important for athletes to consume enough protein to support muscle growth and repair, but it's also important to consume a balanced diet that includes plenty of fruits, vegetables, whole grains, and healthy fats.

Legumes and pulses

Legumes and pulses are a great source of plant-based protein, which is essential for athletes to support muscle repair and growth, as well as aid in recovery after exercise. They are also rich in complex carbohydrates, fiber, vitamins, and minerals, making them an excellent addition to any athlete's diet.

Here are some examples of legumes and pulses that can benefit athletes:

Lentils: Lentils are an excellent source of plant-based protein, fiber, and carbohydrates. They are also rich in iron, which is essential for athletes as it helps transport oxygen to muscles.

Chickpeas: Chickpeas are a good source of protein, fiber, and complex carbohydrates. They are also rich in folate and iron, which are important for energy production and muscle function.

Black beans: Black beans are high in protein, fiber, and complex carbohydrates. They are also rich in antioxidants and potassium, which can help reduce muscle soreness after exercise.

Peas: Peas are a good source of protein, carbohydrates, and fiber. They are also high in vitamin C, which can help support the immune system and reduce inflammation.

Soybeans: Soybeans are a complete source of plant-based protein, containing all nine essential amino acids. They are also high in iron, calcium, and vitamin D, which are important for bone health and muscle function.

Incorporating legumes and pulses into meals such as salads, soups, stews, and curries can provide a well-rounded and nutritious meal for athletes. It's also important to pair them with complex carbohydrates such as whole grains, fruits, and vegetables to provide sustained energy during exercise.

Tofu and tempeh

Tofu and tempeh can be great sources of protein for athletes. Both tofu and tempeh are made from soybeans and are plant-based sources of protein.

Tofu is made by curdling fresh soy milk and then pressing it into a solid block. It is low in fat, high in protein, and contains all nine essential amino acids that are necessary for building and repairing muscles. Tofu is also a good source of iron, calcium, and magnesium.

Tempeh, on the other hand, is made by fermenting cooked soybeans with a specific type of mold. This fermentation process increases the protein and nutrient content of the soybeans, making tempeh an even more nutritious source of plant-based protein. Tempeh is also high in fiber, vitamins, and minerals, including calcium, iron, and zinc.

Both tofu and tempeh can be used in a variety of dishes, including stir-fries, salads, sandwiches, and more. Athletes can benefit from incorporating these plant-based protein sources into their diets to help support muscle growth, repair, and recovery.

Seitan and other wheat-based protein sources

Seitan, also known as wheat meat or wheat gluten, is a popular protein source for athletes who follow a vegetarian or vegan diet. It is made from wheat protein, which is isolated from wheat flour by removing the starch. The resulting product is high in protein, low in fat, and contains all essential amino acids.

Seitan can be prepared in a variety of ways, such as grilling, baking, or frying, and can be flavored with a range of herbs and spices. It can also be used as a meat substitute in recipes such as stir-fries, stews, and sandwiches.

In addition to seitan, there are other wheat-based protein sources that athletes can incorporate into their diet. These include:

Wheat Germ: Wheat germ is the nutrient-rich embryo of the wheat kernel that is removed during the refining process. It is a good source of protein, fiber, and various vitamins and minerals, including vitamin E, which has antioxidant properties that can help reduce muscle damage caused by exercise.

Bulgur: Bulgur is a type of wheat grain that is pre-cooked and dried, making it a quick and easy source of protein for athletes. It is also high in fiber and low in fat, making it a good choice for weight management.

Wheat Berries: Wheat berries are the whole, unprocessed kernels of wheat. They are high in protein, fiber, and various vitamins and minerals, including iron and zinc, which are important for athletes.

It's important to note that some people may have gluten intolerance or celiac disease and should avoid wheat-based protein sources. In such cases, athletes can consider other plant-based protein sources, such as soy, pea, or hemp protein, as well as animal-based sources such as eggs, dairy, and meat.

Plant-based protein powders

Plant-based protein powders can be a great option for athletes who want to supplement their diet with additional protein. Here are some popular plant-based protein powders:

Pea protein powder: Pea protein powder is a popular option for athletes because it is high in protein, with approximately 20-25 grams of protein per serving. It is also easily digestible and contains all of the essential amino acids.

Soy protein powder: Soy protein powder is another popular option for athletes. It is a complete protein, meaning it contains all of the essential amino acids. It is also high in protein, with approximately 20-25 grams of protein per serving.

Brown rice protein powder: Brown rice protein powder is a good option for athletes who are allergic to soy or have other dietary restrictions. It is not a complete protein on its own, but it can be combined with other plant-based protein powders to create a complete protein. It is also easily digestible and contains approximately 20-25 grams of protein per serving.

Hemp protein powder: Hemp protein powder is a good option for athletes who are looking for a plant-based protein powder that also contains other nutrients, such as omega-3 fatty acids and fiber. It is not a complete protein on its own, but it can be combined with other plant-based protein powders to create a complete protein. It contains approximately 10-15 grams of protein per serving.

Pumpkin seed protein powder: Pumpkin seed protein powder is another option for athletes who are looking for a plant-based protein powder that also contains other nutrients, such as magnesium and zinc. It is not a complete protein on its own, but it can be combined with other plant-based protein powders to create a complete protein. It contains approximately 15-20 grams of protein per serving.

When selecting a plant-based protein powder, it is important to look for one that is free of additives, artificial flavors, and sweeteners. It is also important to choose a powder that is certified organic, non-GMO, and third-party tested for purity and quality.

CHAPTER THREE

Plant-Based Carbohydrate Sources for Athletes

Plant-based carbohydrates are an excellent source of energy for athletes. Here are some of the best options:

Whole grains: Whole grains such as brown rice, quinoa, oatmeal, and whole wheat pasta are high in carbohydrates, fiber, and other essential nutrients. They provide a slow, sustained release of energy, making them an excellent choice for endurance athletes.

Fruits: Fruits are rich in carbohydrates, vitamins, minerals, and antioxidants. Bananas, apples, oranges, and berries are great options for athletes. They provide a quick source of energy and can be easily incorporated into pre- or post-workout snacks.

Vegetables: Starchy vegetables such as sweet potatoes, yams, and corn are high in carbohydrates and provide a sustained release of energy. Other non-starchy vegetables such as leafy greens, broccoli, and peppers are also important for athletes as they are rich in vitamins and minerals.

Legumes: Legumes such as lentils, chickpeas, and black beans are a good source of both carbohydrates and protein. They are also rich in fiber, which helps with digestion and promotes feelings of fullness.

Nuts and seeds: Nuts and seeds are a good source of healthy fats, protein, and carbohydrates. They are also rich in vitamins, minerals, and antioxidants. Almonds, cashews, pumpkin seeds, and chia seeds are all great options for athletes.

Overall, incorporating a variety of plant-based carbohydrate sources into an athlete's diet can provide the necessary energy and nutrients needed for optimal performance.

Whole grains

Whole grains are an excellent source of complex carbohydrates, fiber, vitamins, and minerals, making them a great food choice for athletes. They provide sustained energy for physical activity and help maintain a healthy digestive system, among other benefits.

Here are some whole grains that athletes can include in their diet:

Brown rice: Brown rice is a great source of complex carbohydrates, fiber, and B vitamins, making it an excellent food for athletes. It is also a good source of magnesium, which can help regulate muscle and nerve function.

Quinoa: Quinoa is a complete protein, meaning it contains all nine essential amino acids. It is also a great source of complex carbohydrates and fiber, making it an ideal food for athletes.

Oats: Oats are an excellent source of fiber, which can help regulate digestion and keep you feeling full. They are also a good source of complex carbohydrates and B vitamins.

Whole wheat pasta: Whole wheat pasta is a great source of complex carbohydrates, fiber, and B vitamins. It is also a good source of protein and iron, making it an ideal food for athletes.

Barley: Barley is a good source of fiber, complex carbohydrates, and B vitamins. It also contains iron, which is important for oxygen transport to muscles.

Buckwheat: Buckwheat is a good source of protein, fiber, and complex carbohydrates. It is also a great source of magnesium, which can help regulate muscle and nerve function.

Whole grain bread: Whole grain bread is a good source of complex carbohydrates, fiber, and B vitamins. It is also a good source of protein, making it an ideal food for athletes.

Including a variety of these whole grains in your diet can provide sustained energy for physical activity, help regulate digestion, and provide important vitamins and minerals for overall health.

Fruits and vegetables

Fruits and vegetables are an important part of any athlete's diet, as they provide essential vitamins, minerals, fiber, and antioxidants that support overall health and performance. Here are some of the best fruits and vegetables for athletes:

Leafy greens: Leafy greens like spinach, kale, and arugula are packed with vitamins A, C, and K, as well as iron, calcium, and folate. They're also high in nitrates, which can help improve endurance and reduce blood pressure.

Berries: Berries like blueberries, raspberries, and strawberries are high in antioxidants, which can help reduce inflammation and oxidative stress in the body. They're also a good source of fiber and vitamin C.

Citrus fruits: Citrus fruits like oranges, grapefruits, and lemons are high in vitamin C, which is essential for immune function and collagen synthesis. They're also a good source of potassium, which can help regulate blood pressure.

Bananas: Bananas are a great source of carbohydrates, potassium, and vitamin B6, which can help reduce muscle cramps and support energy production.

Sweet potatoes: Sweet potatoes are high in complex carbohydrates, fiber, and vitamin A, which can help support immune function and improve recovery after exercise.

Tomatoes: Tomatoes are high in lycopene, a powerful antioxidant that can help reduce inflammation and oxidative stress. They're also a good source of vitamin C and potassium.

Avocado: Avocado is a good source of healthy fats, fiber, and potassium, which can help support heart health and reduce inflammation.

Broccoli: Broccoli is high in vitamin C, fiber, and sulforaphane, a compound that can help reduce inflammation and improve detoxification.

Remember to include a variety of fruits and vegetables in your diet to ensure you're getting all the essential nutrients your body needs to perform at its best.

Beans and legumes

Beans and legumes are a great source of nutrition for athletes. They are an excellent source of complex carbohydrates, protein, fiber, vitamins, and minerals. Here are some of the benefits of incorporating beans and legumes into an athlete's diet:

High in protein: Beans and legumes are an excellent source of plant-based protein. They contain all essential amino acids required by the body to build and repair muscles, making them an ideal food for athletes.

Carbohydrates: They are also a good source of complex carbohydrates that provide a slow and steady release of energy. This is beneficial for athletes who require sustained energy for their training or competition.

Fiber: Beans and legumes are high in fiber, which helps to promote digestive health and reduce the risk of chronic diseases such as heart disease, diabetes, and some types of cancer.

Vitamins and minerals: Beans and legumes are rich in vitamins and minerals such as iron, zinc, potassium, and B vitamins. These nutrients are essential for maintaining optimal health and performance.

Some examples of beans and legumes that athletes can include in their diet are:

Lentils: Lentils are high in protein, fiber, and complex carbohydrates. They are also a good source of iron, which is essential for carrying oxygen to the muscles.

Chickpeas: Chickpeas are a good source of protein and fiber. They are also high in potassium, which helps to regulate fluid balance in the body.

Black beans: Black beans are a great source of protein, fiber, and complex carbohydrates. They are also high in iron, which is essential for athletes who may be at risk of iron deficiency.

Kidney beans: Kidney beans are high in protein and fiber. They are also a good source of potassium and B vitamins.

Edamame: Edamame are young soybeans that are high in protein, fiber, and complex carbohydrates. They are also a good source of calcium and iron.

Beans and legumes are an excellent source of nutrition for athletes. They provide a range of nutrients that are essential for maintaining optimal health and performance. Including them in the diet can help athletes to achieve their fitness goals and perform at their best.

Sweet potatoes and other root vegetables

Sweet potatoes and other root vegetables can be excellent sources of carbohydrates, vitamins, and minerals for athletes. Carbohydrates are a primary source of energy for athletes, and consuming them before, during, and after exercise can help improve performance and aid in recovery.

Sweet potatoes, in particular, are a great choice for athletes because they are a complex carbohydrate that is low on the glycemic index. This means that they are digested slowly, providing a sustained release of energy that can be particularly useful for endurance athletes. Additionally, sweet potatoes are rich in potassium, which is important for maintaining proper electrolyte balance and preventing muscle cramps.

Other root vegetables that can be beneficial for athletes include beets, carrots, and parsnips. Beets, for example, contain nitrates that can help improve blood flow and oxygen delivery to muscles, potentially enhancing endurance performance. Carrots are high in beta-carotene, which can help support immune function, and parsnips are a good source of folate, which is important for red blood cell production.

Overall, incorporating a variety of root vegetables into an athlete's diet can provide important nutrients and energy to support their performance and recovery.

CHAPTER FOUR

Plant-Based Fat Sources for Athletes

Plant-based diets can be a great option for athletes who are looking to improve their health and performance. There are plenty of plant-based fat sources that can provide athletes with the energy and nutrients they need to excel in their sports. Here are some of the best plant-based fat sources for athletes:

Nuts and Seeds: Nuts and seeds are a great source of healthy fats, protein, and fiber. They are also rich in vitamins and minerals that are important for athletes, such as magnesium, zinc, and vitamin E. Some good options include almonds, walnuts, chia seeds, and flaxseeds.

Avocado: Avocado is a delicious and nutrient-dense fruit that is high in healthy monounsaturated and polyunsaturated fats. It is also a good source of fiber, vitamins, and minerals, such as potassium and vitamin K.

Coconut and Coconut Oil: Coconut and coconut oil are rich in medium-chain triglycerides (MCTs), which are a type of healthy fat that can be quickly absorbed and used for energy. Coconut oil can be used in cooking or baking, while coconut meat and milk can be used in smoothies or as a topping for oatmeal or yogurt.

Olives and Olive Oil: Olives and olive oil are a great source of healthy monounsaturated fats, which can help lower cholesterol levels and reduce the risk of heart disease. Olive oil can be used in cooking, salad dressings, or as a dip for bread.

Tofu and Tempeh: Tofu and tempeh are both made from soybeans and are good sources of healthy fats, protein, and fiber. They are also rich in vitamins and minerals, such as iron and calcium, which are important for athletes.

Dark Chocolate: Dark chocolate is a delicious and nutrient-dense food that is high in healthy fats, antioxidants, and flavonoids. It can be eaten as a snack or used in baking.

Incorporating these plant-based fat sources into a well-balanced diet can help athletes meet their energy and nutrient needs while also improving their health and performance.

Nuts and seeds

Nuts and seeds are an excellent source of nutrition for athletes due to their high content of protein, healthy fats, fiber, vitamins, and minerals. Here are some of the best nuts and seeds for athletes:

Almonds: Almonds are a great source of protein, healthy fats, and fiber. They are also high in vitamin

E, which has been shown to help reduce inflammation and muscle damage.

Walnuts: Walnuts are rich in omega-3 fatty acids, which have been shown to help reduce inflammation and improve heart health. They also contain protein, fiber, and vitamin E.

Pistachios: Pistachios are a good source of protein, fiber, and healthy fats. They also contain potassium, which can help regulate blood pressure and improve heart health.

Chia seeds: Chia seeds are high in protein, fiber, and omega-3 fatty acids. They also contain calcium and magnesium, which are important for bone health.

Flax seeds: Flax seeds are a good source of omega-3 fatty acids, fiber, and lignans, which have been shown to help reduce inflammation and improve heart health.

Pumpkin seeds: Pumpkin seeds are high in protein, healthy fats, and minerals such as magnesium, zinc, and potassium. They also contain antioxidants, which can help reduce inflammation and improve immune function.

Sunflower seeds: Sunflower seeds are a good source of protein, healthy fats, and vitamin E. They also contain minerals such as magnesium and selenium, which are important for muscle and bone health.

When incorporating nuts and seeds into your diet, it's important to keep portion sizes in mind. While they are nutrient-dense foods, they are also calorie-dense, so it's best to eat them in moderation to avoid consuming too many calories.

Avocado

Avocado is a great food choice for athletes as it is packed with essential nutrients that can support athletic performance and recovery.

Healthy fats: Avocado is rich in healthy monounsaturated and polyunsaturated fats which can help improve heart health, regulate cholesterol levels, and reduce inflammation.

Fiber: Avocado is a good source of fiber which can aid in digestion and help regulate blood sugar levels.

Vitamins and minerals: Avocado is a good source of vitamins and minerals including potassium, vitamin K, vitamin C, and vitamin E. These nutrients are essential for muscle function, bone health, and immune function.

Energy: Avocado is a great source of energy due to its high calorie and healthy fat content. It can provide sustained energy for athletes during long workouts or training sessions.

Anti-inflammatory properties: Avocado contains anti-inflammatory compounds such as carotenoids, phytosterols, and flavonoids which can help reduce inflammation and aid in recovery after exercise.

Avocado is a great food choice for athletes due to its nutrient-dense profile and health benefits. It can be enjoyed in a variety of ways such as sliced on toast, blended into smoothies, or added to salads.

Coconut oil and other plant-based oils

Coconut oil and other plant-based oils can be a healthy addition to an athlete's diet when consumed in moderation. They are high in healthy fats, which can provide sustained energy and improve recovery after exercise. Here are some of the benefits and considerations of using coconut oil and other plant-based oils for athletes:

Coconut oil: Coconut oil is a great source of medium-chain triglycerides (MCTs), which are easily digestible and can provide a quick source of energy. It is also high in lauric acid, which has antimicrobial properties that can support immune function. However, coconut oil is also high in saturated fat, so it should be consumed in moderation.

Olive oil: Olive oil is a heart-healthy oil that is high in monounsaturated fats. It can help reduce inflammation and lower the risk of heart disease. It is also rich in antioxidants, which can help protect cells from damage caused by exercise-induced oxidative stress.

Avocado oil: Avocado oil is high in monounsaturated fats and is also a good source of vitamin E, which can help support immune function and reduce inflammation. It can also improve absorption of carotenoids from vegetables, which are important for eye health and immune function.

Flaxseed oil: Flaxseed oil is a great source of omega-3 fatty acids, which are important for brain and heart health. It can also help reduce inflammation and improve insulin sensitivity. However, it is not as stable as other oils and can easily become rancid, so it should be kept refrigerated and used within a few weeks of opening.

When incorporating plant-based oils into an athlete's diet, it's important to consume them in moderation and choose high-quality oils. They can be used for cooking, added to smoothies, or drizzled over salads. It's also important to remember that oils are high in calories, so they should be consumed in appropriate portions based on individual calorie needs.

Vegan margarine and butter substitutes

Here are some general tips for athletes looking for vegan margarine and butter substitutes:

Coconut Oil: This is a popular vegan substitute for butter and margarine in cooking and baking. Coconut oil is rich in medium-chain triglycerides (MCTs), which can provide quick energy to athletes.

Avocado: Avocado can be used as a substitute for butter or margarine in recipes, such as spreads or dips. Avocado is rich in healthy fats, fiber, and potassium, which can help athletes maintain good health.

Nut Butters: Nut butters, such as almond, cashew, or peanut butter, can be used as a spread on toast or as a substitute for butter or margarine in baking. Nut butters are rich in healthy fats, protein, and fiber, which can help athletes maintain good health.

Vegan Margarine: Look for vegan margarines made from plant-based oils, such as sunflower, soybean, or canola oil. These margarines are often fortified with vitamins and minerals and can be used as a substitute for butter in cooking and baking.

Olive Oil: Olive oil can be used as a substitute for butter or margarine in cooking and baking. It is rich in healthy fats and antioxidants, which can help athletes maintain good health.

CHAPTER FIVE

Hydration for Plant-Based Athletes

Hydration is important for all athletes, including plant-based athletes. Proper hydration can improve athletic performance, prevent dehydration and heat-related illnesses, and aid in recovery. Here are some tips for plant-based athletes to stay hydrated:

Drink water regularly: Drinking water is the best way to stay hydrated. Aim to drink water throughout the day, not just during workouts or events. Carry a reusable water bottle with you to ensure that you always have water available.

Eat hydrating foods: Some plant-based foods are naturally high in water content, such as fruits and vegetables. Include these in your diet to help you stay hydrated. Examples include watermelon, cucumber, strawberries, lettuce, and celery.

Use electrolyte replacements: Electrolytes are minerals that help regulate the body's fluid balance. During intense exercise, electrolytes are lost through sweat. Plant-based athletes can use electrolyte replacements such as sports drinks, coconut water, or electrolyte tablets to replenish their electrolyte levels.

Monitor urine color: Urine color can indicate hydration status. Aim for a light, straw-colored urine. Darker urine may indicate dehydration, and colorless urine may indicate overhydration.

Adjust hydration needs based on activity level: Plant-based athletes may have different hydration needs depending on their activity level, sweat rate, and climate. It's important to adjust your hydration plan accordingly. Consult a sports dietitian to help you determine your individual hydration needs.

Staying hydrated is important for all athletes, including plant-based athletes. Drink water regularly, eat hydrating foods, use electrolyte replacements, monitor urine color, and adjust hydration needs based on activity level to ensure proper hydration.

The importance of hydration for athletes

Hydration is crucial for athletes, as it plays a vital role in their performance, recovery, and overall health. Here are some of the reasons why hydration is important for athletes:

Regulates body temperature: When you exercise, your body temperature rises. Sweating is the body's way of cooling down, and the sweat evaporates from your skin to help regulate your body temperature. However, if you're not properly hydrated, you may not be able to produce enough sweat, and your body temperature may rise to dangerous levels, leading to heat exhaustion or heat stroke.

Maintains blood volume: When you exercise, your muscles need more oxygen and nutrients to function. Blood delivers these essential elements to the muscles. But if you're dehydrated, your blood volume decreases, and your heart has to work harder to circulate the blood. This can lead to decreased performance and even fainting.

Prevents cramping: Dehydration can also cause muscle cramps, which can be painful and affect your performance. Cramping occurs when the muscle fibers contract and don't relax, leading to a painful spasm.

Boosts energy levels: When you're dehydrated, your body has to work harder to perform the same tasks. This can lead to fatigue and decreased energy levels, which can affect your performance.

Promotes recovery: After exercise, your body needs to replenish the fluids and nutrients lost during the workout. Adequate hydration can help your body recover faster and reduce the risk of injury or illness.

To ensure proper hydration, athletes should drink plenty of fluids before, during, and after exercise. Water is the best choice for most people, but sports drinks can also be beneficial for athletes who engage in prolonged, intense exercise. It's also important to monitor your urine color and frequency to ensure you're adequately hydrated. If your urine is dark yellow or infrequent, you may need to drink more fluids.

Plant-based sources of hydration

Staying hydrated is crucial for maintaining good health and ensuring that your body functions properly. While water is the most obvious source of hydration, there are also several plant-based foods that can help keep you hydrated. Here are some examples:

Fruits: Fruits are high in water content and can help keep you hydrated. Some of the best fruits for hydration include watermelon, strawberries, oranges, grapefruit, pineapple, and cantaloupe.

Vegetables: Many vegetables are also high in water content and can help keep you hydrated. Some good options include cucumber, celery, lettuce, zucchini, and broccoli.

Soups and stews: Soups and stews are often made with water and can help you stay hydrated. Try vegetable-based soups or broths for a hydrating option.

Smoothies and juices: Smoothies and juices can also be a great source of hydration. Be sure to choose options made with fresh fruits and vegetables, rather than those with added sugars.

Coconut water: Coconut water is a natural source of electrolytes and can be a great way to stay hydrated. It is also low in calories and sugar.

Herbal teas: Herbal teas, such as peppermint or chamomile, can help keep you hydrated and provide other health benefits as well.

Remember to drink plenty of water as well, as it is still the best way to stay hydrated.

Tips for staying hydrated during exercise

Staying hydrated during exercise is essential for maintaining your performance, avoiding fatigue, and preventing dehydration-related health issues. Here are some tips for staying hydrated during exercise:

Drink water before, during, and after exercise: Drink at least 16-20 ounces of water 2-3 hours before exercising and then 8-10 ounces every 10-20 minutes during exercise.

Monitor your urine color: Urine color can be a good indicator of hydration status. Aim for pale yellow to clear urine, indicating you are well hydrated.

Use a sports drink for intense workouts: If you're exercising intensely for more than an hour, a sports drink containing carbohydrates and electrolytes can help replenish lost fluids and electrolytes.

Avoid caffeinated and alcoholic beverages: Caffeine and alcohol are diuretics that can increase urine output and contribute to dehydration. So, it's best to avoid them before and during exercise.

Pay attention to your thirst: Drink water whenever you feel thirsty during exercise.

Consider the environment: If you're exercising in hot or humid conditions, you may need to drink more water to compensate for increased sweating.

Plan ahead: Make sure to bring enough water or sports drinks with you when exercising outdoors or at the gym.

Remember that hydration is crucial for optimal physical performance and overall health. By following these tips, you can help ensure that you stay hydrated during exercise.

CHAPTER SIX

Plant-Based Meal Planning for Athletes

Plant-based diets can be a great way for athletes to fuel their bodies with the necessary nutrients and energy for training and competition. Here are some tips for plant-based meal planning for athletes:

Focus on whole plant foods: Include plenty of fruits, vegetables, whole grains, legumes, nuts, and seeds in your meals. These foods are rich in vitamins, minerals, fiber, and phytonutrients that are important for optimal health and athletic performance.

Get enough protein: Plant-based sources of protein include beans, lentils, chickpeas, tofu, tempeh, nuts, and seeds. Aim for at least 1 gram of protein per kilogram of body weight per day.

Incorporate healthy fats: Nuts, seeds, avocados, and olive oil are great sources of healthy fats that can provide sustained energy for workouts and competitions.

Plan your meals ahead of time: Meal prepping can save time and ensure that you have healthy meals available when you need them. Cook large batches of grains, beans, and vegetables that can be used in multiple meals throughout the week.

Don't forget about hydration: Proper hydration is crucial for athletic performance. Make sure to drink enough water throughout the day, especially before, during, and after workouts.

Consider supplements: Some plant-based athletes may need to supplement with certain nutrients, such as vitamin B12, iron, and omega-3 fatty acids.

Consult with a registered dietitian to determine if you need supplements and how much to take.

Be mindful of calorie intake: Athletes require more calories than sedentary individuals, so make sure you are eating enough to support your training and performance goals.

Experiment with new recipes and flavors: Eating a plant-based diet doesn't have to be boring or bland. Try new recipes and flavor combinations to keep your meals interesting and enjoyable.

Remember to listen to your body and adjust your meal plan as needed to meet your individual needs and preferences. Consult with a registered dietitian who specializes in sports nutrition for personalized recommendations.

Strategies for meal planning on a plant-based diet

Meal planning for athletes on a plant-based diet requires careful attention to ensure that they are getting enough nutrients, calories, and protein to support their athletic performance and recovery. Here are some strategies for meal planning on a plant-based diet for athletes:

Focus on whole, nutrient-dense foods: Incorporate a variety of fruits, vegetables, whole grains, legumes, nuts, and seeds into your meals to ensure you are getting a wide range of vitamins, minerals, and antioxidants. These foods will also provide you with the fiber and carbohydrates you need for energy.

Plan your protein sources: It's important for athletes to consume enough protein to support muscle growth and repair. Good plant-based sources of protein include soy products, legumes, nuts, seeds, and whole grains.

Be sure to include a variety of protein sources in your meals to ensure you are getting all the essential amino acids your body needs.

Incorporate healthy fats: Include healthy fats in your meals to help keep you feeling full and satisfied. Good plant-based sources of healthy fats include avocados, nuts, seeds, olive oil, and coconut oil.

Be mindful of your calorie intake: Athletes on a plant-based diet may need to consume more calories than their omnivorous counterparts to support their athletic performance. Be sure to calculate your daily calorie needs and plan your meals accordingly.

Pre-plan your meals and snacks: Planning your meals and snacks in advance can help ensure you are getting the nutrients and calories you need throughout the day. Meal prepping can also save time and ensure you have healthy options readily available.

Consider nutrient supplementation: While a well-planned plant-based diet can provide all the nutrients you need, some athletes may benefit from supplementing with certain nutrients such as vitamin B12, iron, and omega-3 fatty acids.

Stay hydrated: Hydration is essential for athletes, regardless of their diet. Be sure to drink enough water and consider including hydrating foods such as fruits and vegetables in your meals and snacks.

Overall, meal planning on a plant-based diet for athletes requires careful attention to ensure they are meeting their nutrient and calorie needs. By focusing on whole, nutrient-dense foods and planning meals in advance, athletes can fuel their bodies for optimal performance and recovery.

Sample meal plans for athletes on a plant-based diet

Here are three sample meal plans for athletes on a plant-based diet:

Meal Plan 1:
Breakfast:
Tofu scramble with spinach, tomatoes, and mushrooms
Whole wheat toast with almond butter
Fresh fruit salad

Lunch:
Chickpea salad with mixed greens, avocado, and cherry tomatoes
Baked sweet potato
Hummus and carrots for dipping

Dinner:
Lentil and vegetable stir-fry with brown rice
Steamed broccoli with lemon juice

Mixed berries with vegan yogurt

Snacks:

Protein smoothie with banana, peanut butter, and plant-based protein powder

Handful of mixed nuts

Apple slices with almond butter

Meal Plan 2:

Breakfast:

Vegan protein pancakes with blueberries and maple syrup

Fresh fruit

Soy milk

Lunch:

Quinoa and black bean bowl with avocado, salsa, and mixed greens

Whole wheat pita bread

Roasted chickpeas

Dinner:
Vegan chili with mixed vegetables
Brown rice
Roasted sweet potatoes

Snacks:
Vegan protein bar
Green smoothie with spinach, banana, and almond milk
Rice cakes with hummus

Meal Plan 3:
Breakfast:
Vegan protein oatmeal with banana, cinnamon, and maple syrup
Fresh berries
Soy milk

Lunch:
Vegan burrito bowl with rice, black beans, avocado, and salsa
Baked tortilla chips

Mixed fruit salad

Dinner:

Grilled tofu with mixed vegetables

Baked potato

Vegan Caesar salad

Snacks:

Vegan protein shake with berries, banana, and plant-based protein powder

Raw veggies with vegan ranch dip

Homemade trail mix with nuts and dried fruit

Tips for eating out as a plant-based athlete

As a plant-based athlete, it's important to make sure you are fueling your body with nutrient-dense foods that provide enough protein, carbohydrates, healthy fats, vitamins, and minerals to support your active lifestyle. Here are some tips for eating out:

Do your research: Before you go out to eat, research the restaurant menu to see what options are available for plant-based athletes. Look for dishes that include high-protein plant-based sources such as tofu, tempeh, legumes, and quinoa.

Ask for substitutions: Don't be afraid to ask your server if you can substitute animal products for plant-based options. For example, if a dish comes with cheese, ask if you can replace it with avocado or another healthy fat.

Customize your meal: Many restaurants are happy to customize meals to accommodate dietary preferences. Ask if you can have a salad with extra veggies, or if the chef can prepare a dish without added oils or salt.

Be cautious of hidden ingredients: Some dishes may contain hidden animal products or processed ingredients that are not plant-based.

Ask your server if a dish is made with animal products or if there are any hidden ingredients that you should be aware of.

Stick to whole foods: Whenever possible, choose whole foods like fresh fruits, vegetables, whole grains, and legumes. These are the most nutrient-dense options and will provide your body with the energy it needs to perform at its best.

Don't be afraid to bring your own food: If you're unsure about the options available or if you have specific dietary restrictions, consider bringing your own food. Many restaurants are happy to accommodate and may even offer to heat up your meal for you.

Stay hydrated: Remember to drink plenty of water before, during, and after your meal to stay hydrated and help your body recover from your workouts.

By following these tips, you can enjoy eating out while still maintaining a healthy, plant-based diet that supports your athletic performance.

CHAPTER SEVEN

Plant-Based Supplements for Athletes

Plant-based supplements can be a great addition to an athlete's diet, as they can provide a range of nutrients that are essential for optimal performance and recovery. Here are some plant-based supplements that can be beneficial for athletes:

Creatine: Creatine is a natural substance found in animal products such as meat and fish, but it can also be found in plant-based sources such as spirulina and chlorella. Creatine is known for its ability to enhance strength and power output, making it a popular supplement among athletes.

Beta-Alanine: Beta-alanine is an amino acid that is naturally produced by the body, but it can also be found in plant-based sources such as beets and carnosine-rich vegetables. Beta-alanine is known for its ability to increase muscle endurance and delay fatigue during high-intensity exercise.

Branched-Chain Amino Acids (BCAAs): BCAAs are essential amino acids that are found in protein-rich plant-based sources such as quinoa, lentils, and soybeans. BCAAs are known for their ability to reduce muscle damage and promote muscle protein synthesis, which can aid in muscle recovery and growth.

Iron: Iron is an essential mineral that is important for oxygen transport and energy production. Plant-based sources of iron include dark leafy greens, lentils, and quinoa. Iron supplementation may be beneficial for athletes who are at risk of iron deficiency, such as female athletes or athletes who follow a vegetarian or vegan diet.

Vitamin D: Vitamin D is important for bone health and immune function, and it can also play a role in muscle function and athletic performance.

Plant-based sources of vitamin D include fortified plant milks, mushrooms, and fortified breakfast cereals. Vitamin D supplementation may be beneficial for athletes who have low levels of vitamin D, especially during the winter months when sunlight exposure is limited.

It's important to note that supplements should not be relied upon as a substitute for a balanced diet, and it's always best to consult with a healthcare professional before starting any new supplement regimen.

The role of supplements in a plant-based athlete's diet

Supplements can play a role in a plant-based athlete's diet by helping to ensure they are meeting their nutritional needs. While a well-planned plant-based diet can provide all the necessary nutrients for optimal health and athletic performance, athletes may have increased nutrient requirements and may find it challenging to consume sufficient quantities of certain nutrients solely through their diet.

Here are some supplements that plant-based athletes may consider incorporating into their diet:

Vitamin B12: Vitamin B12 is primarily found in animal products, so plant-based athletes may need to supplement to ensure they are meeting their daily requirements.

Vitamin D: Vitamin D is essential for bone health and can be difficult to obtain through diet alone. Plant-based athletes may need to supplement if they are not getting enough vitamin D from sunlight or fortified foods.

Iron: Plant-based sources of iron may not be as readily absorbed as animal sources, so some athletes may need to supplement to ensure they are meeting their iron needs.

Omega-3s: Plant-based sources of omega-3 fatty acids, such as flaxseeds and chia seeds, may not be as bioavailable as animal sources. Plant-based athletes may consider supplementing with an algae-based omega-3 supplement.

Protein: While most plant-based athletes can meet their protein needs through diet alone, some may benefit from supplementing with a plant-based protein powder to ensure they are meeting their daily requirements.

It's important to note that supplements should not be used to replace whole foods in the diet. Plant-based athletes should focus on consuming a varied and balanced diet that includes a variety of whole plant foods to ensure they are meeting their nutrient needs. It's also important to speak with a healthcare provider or registered dietitian before starting any new supplements to ensure they are safe and appropriate for individual needs.

Key supplements for plant-based athletes

As a plant-based athlete, it's important to ensure that you are getting all the necessary nutrients to support your athletic performance and recovery. While a balanced diet can provide most of the necessary nutrients, some supplements may be beneficial. Here are some key supplements for plant-based athletes:

Vitamin B12: Vitamin B12 is mainly found in animal products and is essential for red blood cell production, nerve function, and DNA synthesis. Plant-based athletes may be at a higher risk of vitamin B12 deficiency, so it's recommended to take a vitamin B12 supplement.

Iron: Iron is important for oxygen transport and energy production. Plant-based athletes may need to consume more iron because plant-based sources of iron are less readily absorbed than animal sources.

An iron supplement can help ensure you are getting enough iron.

Creatine: Creatine is a popular supplement for athletes that may help improve strength, power, and muscle mass. While creatine is mainly found in animal products, it can also be obtained from plant-based sources like creatine supplements made from fermented vegan sources.

Omega-3 fatty acids: Omega-3 fatty acids are important for brain function, heart health, and reducing inflammation. Plant-based sources of omega-3s like flaxseeds, chia seeds, and walnuts are less potent than those found in fish oil. Thus, an omega-3 supplement made from algae is a great option for plant-based athletes.

Protein powder: While it's possible to get enough protein from a plant-based diet, some plant-based athletes may find it challenging to consume enough protein for their needs. A plant-based protein powder can help meet your protein requirements.

It's important to consult with a registered dietitian or healthcare professional before adding any supplements to your diet. They can help determine which supplements you may need and in what dosages.

CONCLUSION

In conclusion, plant-based diets have been shown to be a viable option for athletes looking to optimize their performance and health. By focusing on whole, nutrient-dense foods such as fruits, vegetables, legumes, whole grains, nuts, and seeds, athletes can meet their energy and nutrient needs while also benefiting from the anti-inflammatory, antioxidant, and other health-promoting properties of these foods.

Research has shown that plant-based diets can provide sufficient protein, carbohydrate, fat, and other key nutrients to support athletic performance, and may even offer advantages over animal-based diets in terms of improving cardiovascular health, reducing inflammation, and enhancing recovery from exercise-induced muscle damage.

However, it is important for athletes to work with a registered dietitian or other qualified nutrition professional to ensure they are meeting their individual nutrient needs and fueling properly for their sport. Athletes should also consider factors such as taste preferences, cultural and social factors, and practicality when making dietary changes.

Overall, a well-planned plant-based diet can be a healthy and effective option for athletes, and may offer benefits beyond just improving athletic performance.

Printed in Great Britain
by Amazon

22755895R00050